Table of Contents

Understanding Multiple Food Allergies (MFA)

1. Introduction to Multiple Food Allergies (MFA)

2. Prevalence and Incidence of Multiple Food Allergies

3. Types of Multiple Food Allergies

3.1. Cross-Reactivity

3.2. Co-Sensitization

4. Common Symptoms of Multiple Food Allergies

5. Diagnosis of Multiple Food Allergies

5.1. Skin Prick Test

5.2. Blood Tests

5.3. Oral Food Challenge

Understanding Multiple Food Allergies: Symptoms, Causes, and Management

1. Introduction to Multiple Food Allergies

As parents, carers, and students today are becoming more and more interested in what they put in their body, the subject of multiple food allergies is becoming increasingly important as individuals would like to know possible symptoms that might occur in case of an allergic reaction. Likewise, corporations and charities would have an interest in an associate's job title, and parents would also have an interest in learning how to manage multiple food allergies.

Multiple food allergies are the presence of two or more distinct allergies to food or drink, of which an allergic reaction or severe allergic reaction can occur in single food-allergic individuals. A severe allergic reaction affecting someone with multiple food allergies is called a multiphasic reaction. Multiphasic reactions occur in 2% to 3% of severe allergic reactions where hospitalization or emergency treatment is required, and often sustained ingestion with one or more causal allergens is responsible. Many of the symptoms of multiple food allergies that involve the nervous system may occur in late reactions.

There are multiple types of food allergies that affect individuals. A growing area of research interest is the extent of those who suffer from multiple food allergies. This essay serves to explore what multiple food allergies are, the symptoms involved, the causes of the condition, and how it's best managed.

1. Introduction to Multiple Food Allergies

As parents, carers, and students today are becoming more and more interested in what they put in their body, the subject of multiple food allergies is becoming increasingly important as individuals would like to know possible symptoms that might occur in case of an allergic reaction. Likewise, corporations and charities would have an interest in an associate's job title, and parents would also have an interest in learning how to manage multiple food allergies.

Multiple food allergies are the presence of two or more distinct allergies to food or drink, of which an allergic reaction or severe allergic reaction can occur in single food-allergic individuals. A severe allergic reaction affecting someone with multiple food allergies is called a multiphasic reaction. Multiphasic reactions occur in 2% to 3% of severe allergic reactions where hospitalization or emergency treatment is required, and often sustained ingestion with one or more causal allergens is responsible. Many of the symptoms of multiple food allergies that involve the nervous system may occur in late reactions.

There are multiple types of food allergies that affect individuals. A growing area of research interest is the extent of those who suffer from multiple food allergies. This essay serves to explore what multiple food allergies are, the symptoms involved, the causes of the condition, and how it's best managed.

2. The Immune System and Food Allergies

In at-risk neonates, breastfeeding may help to prevent messy and atopic dermatitis, but it still could lead to many food allergens passing from mother to child. In these cases, mothers will note that they must be screened for likely allergies if they, too, are allergic to a food. An avoidance diet for the food that causes the reaction is generally the main therapy for people with food allergies. Experiment with other medical options because they are regularly changing and are not uniformly disseminated.

As the immune system responds to a particular protein of a food, an allergic reaction can occur, potentially worsening into a more threatening systemic response. Food allergies often materialize in early infancy, and in some cases, these initial and apparently mild reactions build up to more severe and potentially fatal reactions as the immune systems mature. However, some people can develop food allergies in adulthood. Trigger types can also change over time, with one food allergy (e.g., egg) possibly being outgrown and replaced by another (e.g., pollen) in some cases.

Along with the skin and epithelial layers of the respiratory system, the mucosal lining of the gastrointestinal tract separates us from our surrounding environment. The gut associates with the highest number of immune-active cells and is estimated to contain approximately 80% of all lymphocytes in the body. Here, allergens need to be tolerated, keeping in mind that allergens are often proteins and rapidly digested or deteriorated by cooking, making them more accessible by immune surveillance. In some situations, the immune system may react to these harmless, typically likely removed, allergens and defend the body as if they were harmful germs.

The human body is equipped with a specialized set of defenses against harmful pathogens called the immune system. Generally, immune responses are deployed when potentially infectious agents, like bacteria or viruses, are encountered. The way the immune system reacts is finely tuned to eliminate these threats as well as to initiate healing and recovery after the threat is neutralized. Therefore, when working normally, the immune system remains quiet inside most of us, not reacting to substances commonly found in our environment.

2.1. How Food Allergies Develop

Although multiple food allergies have been on the rise in recent years, much research is still needed to better understand most aspects behind their development. Food allergy is a complex disorder and can be related to other "atopic" or allergic diseases such as eczema (atopic dermatitis) and allergic rhinitis (nasal symptoms) as well as "non-atopic" diseases such as celiac disease, an immune reaction to gluten in the diet. Genetics can predispose individuals to have immune reactivity to other environmental allergens and increase the risk for multiple food allergies. Hormonal changes as well as infections in the gastrointestinal tract during infancy have also been linked with an increased number of food allergies. The intestinal and skin barriers perform the same function, namely a physical barrier as well as components within that have the job of neutralizing pathogens before they can do harm.

Just like any other food allergic reaction, when someone is allergic to multiple foods, the immune system mounts an allergic response to certain proteins found in food. It is not really understood why some proteins and not others are capable of inducing these responses that result in allergies. Scientists have investigated sensitization to food that occurs through the skin of young infants with a condition called atopic dermatitis. When proteins in food are applied to the skin over a chronic period of time, the injured skin can more readily have an immune response to food proteins that are deposited on injured skin. Soon thereafter, when the infant ingests these food allergens, an allergic reaction occurs, establishing food allergy. Other research is focusing on how the immune system is skewed away from becoming tolerized to various environmental allergens and how the immune response becomes associated with atopy, or allergic disease.

3. Common Symptoms of Multiple Food Allergies

In the majority of cases, those who suffer from multiple food allergies react to two or more items within the same food domain (e.g. "profiles of allergy to Artemisia" may include one or more of the foods apple, orange, cherry, strawberry, or kiwi; allergy to birch may include peach, apple, pear, or apricot), or to related molecules derived from plant foods: for example, lipid-transfer proteins (LTP), Profilins, or Bet V1-like molecules, among others. In summary, symptoms of multiple types of food allergy can widely vary from individual to individual but commonly affect the digestive system as well as respiratory and skin, with a few in some cases having systemic and severe reactions including anaphylaxis. In adults, multiple food allergy can be associated with severe reactions including anaphylaxis in about 35%, in children this figure is much lower at about 6%.

1. Digestive symptoms can include vomiting, stomach cramps, and diarrhea or loose stools. In some cases, more chronic GI symptoms may mimic food intolerances vs. allergies. 2. Respiratory symptoms may include sneezing, wheezing, and coughing, which can also be caused by viral infections, as part of asthma or provoked by other allergens such as animal dander and pollen. 3. Skin reactions can result in hives and red-rash like blotches. 4. Systemic responses can cause a drop in blood pressure, also known as anaphylaxis.

These symptoms can widely differ and go over and beyond those of single food allergies:

3.1. Digestive Symptoms

Patterns: Due to the complexity of this topic, a commonly accepted definition or classification of "multiple food allergies" at a cellular, molecular, or genetic level does not yet exist. In principle, allergic (IgE-mediated) and non-allergic (cellular-mediated) mechanisms can be divided into two groups. Dietary avoidance can be influenced by the known and unknown risks about diet choice and complications caused by nutritional deficiencies. In clinical practice, the term multiple food allergies or multi-IGE mediated allergies remains applicable here to a wide range of patients.

3.1. Digestive Symptoms Digestive symptoms: Organ systems, main signs and symptoms, gut contents involved Most of the literature exploring signs and symptoms of individuals dealing with multiple food allergies is limited to symptoms affecting the digestive system, emphasizing the importance of this body system in patients affected with multiple food allergies. The main (subjective) symptoms described following the ingestion of a food allergen mainly involve the gastrointestinal (GI) tract. It can range from nausea to diarrhea, hypotension, asthma, abdominal pain, or even anaphylactic reactions. Due to the various symptoms influencing the GI tract and the different pathophysiological pathways, affected patients need an interdisciplinary team of gastroenterologists, allergologists, nutritionists, psychologists, and nursing personnel already being trained in this field.

Multiple food allergies can affect various bodily systems, and the mechanisms of multiple food allergies can be complex and multifaceted. This article aims to provide detailed guidance on understanding the impact of multiple food allergies on individuals, aspects of this condition that define it, and what can be done for treatment and management. Aspects of digestive symptoms are separated further, and then assessment and management.

3.2. Respiratory Symptoms

Rhinitis is characterized by an itchy nose and eyes, sneezing, and watery rhinorrhea. Conjunctivitis is characterized by redness and eye tearing. Food-induced rhinitis and conjunctivitis symptoms are generally mild, and their manifestations depend on the inhalation-eating habits of the person. Bronchospasm is a sudden contraction of the muscles in the wall of the bronchioles in the lower respiratory system, which results in their constriction, leading to difficulty in breathing caused by muscles around the airways tightening, inflammation, and a buildup of thick mucus in the airways. This leads to coughing, wheezing, and shortness of breath, and the rate at which these effects occur is fast when compared to allergen ingestion-associated symptoms. Exercise bronchoconstriction can be a response to the consumption of an allergic food where the threshold and mechanisms differ between individuals.

Food allergy can induce various allergic responses that involve the respiratory system. Rhinitis (inflammation of the lining of the nose) may occur on its own or in combination with conjunctivitis (inflammation of the white part of the eye), known as allergic (or rhinoconjunctivitis). When the allergic response of the naso-bronchioles is activated, it can lead to asthma. These outcome manifestations of food allergy do not normally require the ingestion of food and are typically induced by the inhalation of food proteins.

3.3. Skin Reactions

Dermatologic symptoms of food allergies, especially in cases of multiple food allergens, can be extensive and varied. Skin contact with food can lead to allergic contact dermatitis, typically leading to manifest a site-specific skin irritation within 24-48 h. Despite the borderline clinical relevance based on evidence, a number of allergists and children's hospitals counsel parents to have their children with allergies carry medical stopwatches to avoid waiting for allergic reactions at the allergists' offices. Skin prick tests or atopic patch testing can be diagnostic studies to understand which allergen(s) may be causing contact dermatitis. Local antihistamine cream(s) and systemic antihistamines in a limited number of individuals may be useful for avoidance of the limited patch testing list foods.

Although skin reactions represent one of the four primary medical domains for food allergy (alongside the GI, respiratory, and cardiovascular systems), they can also be a sign of systemic, multi-system allergic reaction. Given the complexity of allergic skin symptoms and mechanisms, as well as the small array of physical and functional symptoms in general, there is a tendency to underappreciate the extent of the dysfunction occurring within elicited allergic reactions. Proper evaluation of allergic skin reactions is a necessary element of diagnosis in any patient identifying with multiple concurrent food allergies, to better understand the natural disease patterns and evaluate those at higher risk of severe, life-threatening allergic reactions. Skin allergy changes, especially hives (urticaria) and swelling (angioedema), are some of the most common reactions in those with multiple food allergies, but are generally more transient and potentially safely managed with the use of antihistamines (i.e., no cardinal vital sign change or need for Epinephrine use).

4. Diagnosis of Multiple Food Allergies

There are proper diagnostic clinical pathways proposed by NICE in 2011. Basically, all the allergic diseases, including food allergies, are diagnosed with a proper clinical history to confirm the diagnosis of a food allergy. Some of the allergy tests include food diaries, skin prick tests using allergens, blood samples for allergen-specific serum IgE, atopy patch tests, and oral food challenge. Based on the results of those tests, a person is managed accordingly. If the results are negative, the person will be encouraged to intake the food allergen. If the food allergen is positive with any of the tests, the person will be placed on an absence of food allergen diet. The clinical pathways help in identifying, managing, and treating the patient without any complications.

Currently, there are no proper protocols for the diagnosis of a multiple food allergy. Progression, one after another, with a proper history of the patient depicting symptoms when accidentally ingesting the offending food, is the best procedure for diagnosing food allergies. Just because the foods are avoided, both current and previous, does not mean that person is allergic to that food. In health, food allergens may change over time, to which a person has become sensitive. Proper follow-up testing of suspected food allergens may be needed over time. Skin prick tests and specific food IgE allergen tests are necessary to prove that a person is allergic to a food. They are important to confirm food allergy and not to start proper management.

4.1. Skin Prick Test

Skin prick test (SPT) SPT is the most frequently used investigative technique to diagnose FA, as small quantities of different allergens can be introduced into the skin quickly and safely. A positive SPT can indicate that a subject has serum IgE antibodies responsive to a specific food and is consistent with clinical manifestations or symptoms suggesting underlying IgE-mediated FA. In addition to facilitating the choice for foods for subsequent diagnostic challenges, identification of the offending food allergen early following detailed clinical history can be beneficial to the quality of life of food allergic patients. The highly accurate identification of the "true" food allergen is important in those individuals with food allergies so that unnecessary dietary restrictions are not placed on the diet; for example, in a baby with a suspected FA, it is important to diagnose cow's milk contact urticaria caused by the gut-derived histamine from the mother's breastmilk rather than labeled "cow's milk allergy". Several different standards of interpretation can be found in the literature which may impact the reproducibility of SPT results. have attempted to establish a single positive threshold for a positive SPT from a systematic review of previously published studies. They suggested that SPT wheal diameters equal or more than 3, 9, and 13 mm should allow a certain and proportional conclusion of a positive predictive value of an FA in epidemiological study, clinical services, and specialist clinics, respectively. A SPT is interpreted by comparing the diameter of the wheal with that of the surrounding flare. If the wheal is found to be the same size as the flare, then this indicates that a positive SPT against the allergen. Generally, the SPTs are considered clinically significant in nonatopic children if the wheal is larger than 3 mm or in atopic children if the wheal is larger than 5 mm. A larger wheal diameter generally correlates with a larger amount of IgE toward the tested allergen.

4.2. Blood Test

Overall, a food allergy diagnosis can be hectic, consisting of endless rounds of tests and can require time and dedication to properly diagnose multiple allergies. Additionally, some tests can cause more harm than good. For example, tests completed in an environmental state (where all body and blood samples are not native to the same country in which the test is performed) may not accurately diagnose true food allergies, while others may cause fear to falsely diagnosed parents and children. Although more research is needed, some laboratories are beginning to incorporate these technologies and tests to determine the presence and severity of multiple food allergies. Above all, it is important to pay attention to the history of reactions and seek help from a professional, rather than relying solely on their expertise.

The blood test, also known as the allergen-specific immunoglobulin E test, is another way to diagnose food allergies. The process returns negative results for those without allergens in their bodies, providing more information to healthcare professionals so that they can diagnose multiple food allergies. These blood tests require that three blood samples from three different patients be placed on the same allergen-specific IgE test surface. In layman's terms, if three blood samples match, an allergic reaction is present. These surfaces contain up to 50 different allergens, however some children can have allergic sensitivities to over a hundred different allergens. Therefore, a blood test would have to compare a large number of different blood samples to evaluate multiple food allergies, which proves to be a lengthy, time-consuming, and expensive process. Additionally, these tests are not available in many countries, making it difficult to conduct widespread research on their abilities to cover various food allergens.

5. Common Food Allergens

1. Peanuts: People with peanut allergies must avoid peanuts and peanut products. Peanuts can cause severe allergic reactions, so airlines, schools, and other public places often restrict peanut consumption. 2. Tree nuts: Almonds, walnuts, cashews, and macadamia are some examples of tree nuts. Each person with a tree nut allergy may have to avoid these tree nuts only or additional tree nuts not mentioned; a healthcare provider should provide guidance on dietary restrictions. 3. Milk: Cow's milk and products made with milk should be avoided by people with cow's milk allergy. Dairy can be included in nearly every processed food, so it can be a challenging allergy to manage. People allergic to cow's milk can sometimes tolerate milk from other animals, such as goats or camels, but the only way to find out is to take part in a food challenge under the care of an allergy specialist.

The allergies to specific foods can affect people of all ages, though children are most likely to develop them. The most common food allergens, which can affect as many as 32 million people in the United States, are peanuts, tree nuts, eggs, milk, wheat, soy, fish, and crustacean shellfish. The good news is that the U.S. Food and Drug Administration (FDA) has mandated that these eight foods must be identified on food labels. It is essential to recognize the signs and symptoms of these common food allergens so people can avoid them and get help if they do encounter these foods.

5.1. Peanuts

A 3 mg dose of peanut protein contains enough peanut allergens to cause a clinical reaction in the most sensitive peanut-allergic patients. Peanut is a hardy allergen which retains its allergenic properties even when fried or frozen. The allergenicity of peanuts is not decreased by being processed with or having contact with or is contaminated with other foods. Consequently, the peanut vulgaris (ground/goober/gravel/earth nut), when processed with other foods and edible materials, retains its identity for the production of labeling standard allergen in composite food products, or as a significant contaminant in food products.

Peanuts are one of the most common food allergens and have significant allergenic properties. It is difficult to identify peanuts in a diet as they are used in a vast array of food products. It is estimated that less than 20% of children with a peanut allergy will outgrow it, and they often retain this type of food allergy into adulthood. Reactions to peanuts can be triggered by the ingestion of minute amounts of peanut protein. Peanut allergy symptoms can range from moderate to severe, with the most common being urticaria (hives), angioedema (swelling), rhinoconjunctivitis, abdominal pain and emesis, diarrhea, and wheeze. The most severe reaction is anaphylaxis, which can become fatal: around 80% of all peanut-induced anaphylaxis results in death.

5.2. Tree Nuts

Adverse reactions to the ingestion of tree nuts are known to be an important cause of allergy, which explains why these foods figure in the "The Big Eight" group of allergens. In general, the symptoms related to tree nut allergy can be classified as an immediate-type (IgE/antibody-mediated) or a non-immediate-type (T cell/delayed type). With respect to tree nut allergy, the former is more frequent and manifests as type I hypersensitivity (urticaria, angioedema, eczema, rhinitis, asthma, wheeze, (abdominal) pain, vomiting, and anaphylaxis). The outgrown age in tree nut allergies range between 3 to 8 years, with peanut and tree nut allergies being outgrown last. The allergic reactions range from mild to life-threatening. Management of tree nut allergy includes vigilance in checking processed foods, restaurant foods, and other foods in the diet. Legumes and fruits are more important for tree nut-allergic consumers than are other tree nuts.

Tree nuts are an important source of nutrients and health benefits, but they are also one of the most common food allergens. Several tree nut proteins are responsible for allergic reactions, with most being storage proteins accountable for the cross-sensitivity observed within this group. Allergic reactions affect the skin, causing acute urticaria or general itching to systemic symptoms that can lead to anaphylaxis. Moreover, many allergens have been described as more than one type of food, i.e., as vegetal food allergens in general or as tree nut allergens.

5.3. Milk

The symptoms of a milk protein allergy are the same as food allergies. Someone who is having a severe allergic reaction to milk may have trouble breathing, talking, or swallowing because of mouth and airway swelling. People with a milk allergy are also more likely to develop allergies to other foods, allergic rhinitis, and asthma. The good news for many children is that they generally outgrow this problem. However, relapse rates are higher in children who are allergic to several foods. Although cow milk and goat milk have many of the same proteins, some people are allergic to cow milk but they are okay with goat milk.

Symptoms of a Milk Allergy

The components of cow's milk responsible for allergic symptoms are proteins, including αS1-casein, β-casein, κ-casein, and β-lactoglobulin. As mentioned for other foods related in this chapter, symptoms occur after the milk protein triggers the immune system and numerous cells, mediators, and cytokines and chemokines are released to activate the allergic reaction. The symptoms of milk allergy are varied and usually occur, involving more than one body system and affecting the skin, respiratory, and gastrointestinal systems. As for other foods problems, the mildest allergy symptoms are the result of a local reaction (such as hives on the skin), while the most severe allergic symptoms are due to life-threatening systemic reaction called anaphylaxis. Milk proteins are most commonly found in milk, but they are also found in foods, such as baked goods, and other products that use dairy products. Moreover, milk is sometimes used to ferment products, like cheese or yogurt. Proteins from these fermented products sometimes cause allergic reactions, but the proteins in baked goods and fermented products.

Allergic Responses

6. Understanding Cross-Reactivity

For example, people allergic to peanuts often develop allergies to at least one of the following: soy (which is actually a legume), black-eyed peas, azuki beans (also called red mung or vani), lentils, chickpeas, and fenugreek. As mentioned previously, seeds belong to the same family as peanuts. Studies have shown that people who test positive for peanut allergy will sometimes test positive on skin-prick tests for other legumes, such as lentils, as well. And, it has been shown that out of 21 children with known peanut allergies, 16 also tested positive for soy allergies. In fact, there is a series of food allergies known as the "peanut-free nut" allergies, as people who are allergic to peanuts can also be allergic to at least one (and usually more) of these nuts: almonds, walnuts, Brazil nuts, cashews, macadamias, pecans, filberts (hazelnuts), pistachios, and ground nuts (peanuts). However, it is not known if these other allergies in those with nut and peanut allergies are the result of a true cross-reactivity or if they are due to the fact that children with allergies to peanuts and nuts tend to be more likely to develop other food allergies.

Cross-reactivity is a phenomenon where proteins in closely related foods are similar enough that the immune system recognizes them all as being the same, even when they come from different sources. Therefore, an individual who is allergic to a certain pollen, for example, may have allergic symptoms when he eats a food that has one of its proteins in common with this pollen, without being allergic to the food. This is a concept that is important to understand for those people who have different known allergies to foods that are closely related.

7. Management of Multiple Food Allergies

People with multiple food allergies can become part of a community of others who are facing and coping with the challenges of this situation. Sharing information and experiences about food management and daily challenges can provide new ideas and help people learn new and different approaches to handling it. Depending on the tools available through support programs and organizations within your community, you have the opportunity to meet and connect with others facing multiple food allergies and to share information and experiences. Since these groups change over time, further information can be obtained from your general medical practitioner. Some of the risk of eating outside the home can be reduced by informing your child's teachers of multiple food allergies, and by discussing ways to recognize and handle severe reactions.

If a person is allergic to at least two foods, this significantly increases the chances of having a reaction. In most cases, avoidance of the allergens responsible is the most effective strategy for preventing allergic reactions in people with multiple food allergies. Careful and cautious home meal preparation can prevent reactions to multiple triggers, and starting new allergy foods can be much more dangerous when there are already several allergies. Although it can be complicated, avoiding foods is an effective way to manage multiple food allergies. Proactive avoidance of food triggers by increasing your knowledge of where potential food allergens can be found and developing label reading skills will help you avoid being exposed to food triggers. Educate yourself about ingredient names known to indicate an allergenic food in one of your allergies. The more information you have, the safer and more comfortable you will be in avoiding your allergic food.

However, food avoidance alone may not necessarily prevent allergic reactions. For people who have had multiple food challenges, it is possible that undiagnosed or masked allergies may be present. These can arise from foods which are allergic to other foods, for example, wheat allergy sufferers sometimes also have to avoid soya; or complex 'cross-reacting' allergies where proteins in different foods all react with the same IgE in an allergic response. These are encountered most often by people with peanut and tree nut allergies. Furthermore, current research suggests, for some people, continued avoidance may lead to a reduction of symptoms and even tolerance for some allergens. Evidence for this was published in the Allergen Bubble project, following a dairy milk food challenge. However, such studies are ongoing and potentially risky, so should only be performed as part of a supervised medical study.

The most effective treatment for multiple food allergies is to avoid all those foods that an individual is allergic to. It is imperative that these foods are removed from the individual's diet and substituted with nutritious, non-allergenic foods, in order to maintain a healthy lifestyle. It is also vital that these foods are avoided in the event of accidental or unintentional exposure.

7.2. Reading Food Labels

In Canada, all foods that come in a package must indicate at the end or side of the ingredient lists if they contain any of the top 11 food allergens. These allergens are (in decreasing order of prevalence) milk, eggs, peanuts, tree nuts, wheat/gluten, soy, sesame, seafood, sulphites, and mustard. Most will indicate if the product "may contain" the allergen due to cross-contamination, but many of us have a no tolerance approach. Additionally, there is no legislation for products sold by individuals or in-person at small businesses (there is different legislation if you sell online or directly to consumers through mail/in-person). Always ask these businesses exactly what is in their product. Always read the entire label, including the allergen statement, as some things derived from potential allergens or present as part of a company's flavorings/starches/similar will be in the ingredients.

Reading labels is essential when you have multiple food allergies, especially when you rely on packaged/pre-made products regularly. As an adult with multiple food allergies, one of my most useful skills is reading and understanding food labels. I often look at labels and form a hypothesis about the contraindicated allergens based on the ingredients; this allows me to predict which products I can't eat without touching them or asking the staff. Label reading is a skill that I strongly advise you to develop because it will make your life exponentially easier.

The practice of reading labels

8. Emergency Response Plan

Keep written instructions at school or in a daycare setting on how to manage an allergic reaction. Before your child enters either a daycare or school, request a meeting with the school nurse and/or appropriate staff to discuss in detail the potential problems this condition may present. Provide emergency medications to your school or daycare setting. Be sure all the medication sent to school is specifically labeled with your child's name, the name of the medication, expired date, dose, frequency, and route of administration. Further, have your physician specify at what point the emergency medications can be administered, and what dosage should be given. Have the school or daycare personnel be able to recognize the signs and symptoms of an allergic reaction in the event your child becomes exposed to a known food allergen at school. A minimum critical level of protein exposure to cause food allergy symptoms is needed before administration of the medication. Plan how the emergency medications and supplies will be stored and readily available if needed.

Have an emergency response plan. No matter how careful your family may be in taking precautions to avoid common food allergens, there may come a time when accidental exposure to a highly allergic trigger will occur. The emergency care plan should be clearly outlined and well defined to let appropriate adults and emergency workers know how to manage an unexpected, yet life-threatening allergic reaction that may occur in your child. The basics to cover are to confirm the diagnosis of anaphylaxis, being prepared, avoid the food, and to know how to recognize allergic reactions.

9. Impact on Quality of Life

Ultimately, the primary issue when managing multiple food allergies from this condition arises from the necessity to manage for coexisting allergies and the limited available food options. Therefore, the feeling of sufficiency and satisfaction with the aforementioned management and the overlap connection fail to satisfy the emotional, social, and medical well-being and the quality of life. These types of individual centers are places where food allergies are often diagnosed or referred to after symptoms present. In the case of food allergy diagnosis, a visit to these centers is essential to manage the combination food allergy while also treating the primary allergy. It is here in these types of doctor's offices and similar patient care centers that management of one will directly affect the treatment of the other.

Chronic conditions, including multiple food allergies, have been shown to have a significant impact on a person's quality of life. The physical symptoms and medical management are often complemented by an emotional burden, such as guilt, worry, and social isolation. Food allergy requires constant vigilance and monitoring to identify and prevent allergic reactions. Research has shown that parents of children with IgE-mediated food allergy report a feeling of guilt, are likely to avoid others, and to bring safe foods to parties. Adults diagnosed with food allergies report episodes of anxiety and hypervigilance when out in public and always double-checking if a meal is safe to eat. Therefore, food allergy carries a psychosocial burden that can be life-shaping. Asthma and food allergy status have shown to be negatively correlated to quality of life. The management of food allergy requires extensive logistical management, time, and attention to prevent allergen exposure.

10. Current Research and Future Directions

Meaningful thresholds to diagnose clinically important multiple food allergies need to be derived. In time, studies such as the Bamba cohort will provide valuable data on allergen exposure resulting from both diet and the environment. Existing studies into allergy to cow's milk may prove useful in understanding how children manage extensive milk allergy and in identifying factors associated with favorable outcomes. In both time windows of introduction to this paper, robust and relevant evidence for the approach to and management of multiple food allergies in childhood does not exist.

This area of research is rapidly expanding, and it's possible that future work will yield a consensus definition of multiple IgE-mediated food allergy. To date, studies largely characterize and describe the allergic population affected. Future work should aim to understand better the mechanisms associated with multiple food allergies and the impact of these complex allergies on quality of life and resource utilization. Descriptive longitudinal summaries and evidence relating to maternal or infant diet from current ongoing studies in general food allergy, 1, 3, 7 nonimmediate presentations of food allergy, 4, 5 nonanaphylactic presentations of food allergy, 9, 34 and non-IgE-mediated presentations are expected to contribute to our understanding.

11. Conclusion and Key Takeaways

Compared with single allergies, it is more prone to secondary complications, making management very difficult. Generally, pharmacological treatment and allergen avoidance are the main management methods, while immunotherapy is a relatively controversial treatment. Several preventive measures can reduce the growth of immunoglobulin E in the body and then weaken the body's reaction. For a person with a food allergy, even though there is a particular treatment, such as strict diet management or a drug that reduces the symptoms of an allergic reaction, several important things must be considered during the treatment process. Many studies have been developed related to treatment combined with hypoallergenic food, which can avoid an allergic reaction after ingesting food.

Multiple food allergies often surface early in life. The symptoms of multiple food allergies are closely related to the individual foods, and the effect on infants and children can lead to severe developmental or psychological problems. When a food allergy occurs, the body's immune system responds as if the individual is being harmed by the allergen. More than 170 foods have been identified as causing food allergies, but not all of them trigger an acute allergic reaction. The most common clinical symptoms are asthma and eczema and, at worst, anaphylaxis. The mechanism of multiple food allergies occurring at the same time is not yet clear, and it is often related to a combination of genetic factors, the type of food and dose, and exposure patterns that affect individual demographics, such as age, ethnicity, location, or social aspects.

Understanding Multiple Food Allergies (MFA)

1. Introduction to Multiple Food Allergies (MFA)

Clearly, more research is needed on what constitutes MFA, how big a problem this represents, and what is the best way to manage such children and their families. There is interest, therefore, in conducting research in collaboration with the top tertiary allergy services in Australia and New Zealand through the AusYAC (Australian and New Zealand Young Adults with Severe Allergic Disease) centres, to address the important public health problem of understanding who suffers from true MFA. Furthermore, little is known about the prevalence and clinical outcomes for adults with severe MFA. Taken together, the main aims of this research are to answer the following questions: 1. What is the current prevalence of MFA in pediatric and adult populations in Australia and how does this differ from the general populations (Australian and NZ)? 2. What is the cost (quality of life) for individuals over time with MFA at baseline? 3. How does management impact on costs (quality of life) of individuals with MFA over time? The findings of this research program will be new knowledge about MFA, for adults and children, which can then guide the allocation of future resources.

It has recently been reported that there is a high prevalence of multiple food allergies (MFA) within the general population. However, what constitutes true multiple food allergies, as opposed to multiple foods believed to cause allergic symptoms, is still a contentious issue. There have been reports of allergies to many different foods, but the overall prevalence of 5 or more allergies has been calculated to be 1.4%-2.5% in Australian children and Icelandic adults (depending on the definition used) using systematic allergy testing followed by food challenges. There are many reports of children with at least 5, or even 10 or more food allergies in the published English literature.

Understanding Multiple Food Allergies (MFA)

2. Prevalence and Incidence of Multiple Food Allergies

The first epidemiological study of food allergy in the infantile patient population surviving beyond the first 12 months of life validated a two-tier diagnostic system that still carries guidelines for practitioners worldwide. At the moment of manuscript submission, serum specific IgE testing with the commonly accepted clinical decision points involving the most allergenic food was the standard diagnostic, with the additional gold standard of the double-blind placebo-controlled food challenge.

Determining the extent of multiple food allergies (MFA) is a daunting task and the numbers vary greatly by age, region, and demographic. It has been observed that MFA can range from 1 in 40 (2.5%) in the general United States' populace to 10-12% of patients visiting allergy clinics. The number of years since MFA diagnosis shows no correlation to the number of foods a patient suffers from, indicating that MFA can occur at any point in a person's life. Epinephrine auto-injectors are a key tool in MFA management and having to carry multiple auto-injectors ups the expense and increases the likelihood of misuse. Patients with multiple allergies typically possess little cataloged empirical data on this condition. This is evidenced by the few published papers on the multifaceted domain of MFA. Education is a key element for any persons suffering from MFA, as well as the medical staff and allies who support the patients.

3. Types of Multiple Food Allergies

The former two types are not the focus of this review. Cross-sensitization and co-sensitization in the case of MAA are not due to similar protein structure, but because of the absorption of stress-hormone adducts of each respective FA-allergenic proteins in each other or in other foods co-consumed along with them. This leads to mounting a multifactorial and individual-specific allergic response. Because the MAA mechanism has multiple allergic response-causative food allergens proceeding through distinct pathways, with many different immune cells and mediators, the symptoms could be multisystemic, with varied and even opposite symptoms that a single food allergy cannot cause. Furthermore, the symptoms often occur only after three days of a pathognomonic meal. It can be recommended that "multiple food allergies due to common allergenic embedded-stress" be termed metabolic-allergy towards multiple foods, and those allergenic additives as metabolic allergens.

Secondly, MAA is suggested, irrespective of whether the individual partakes in FA or not. This occurs in individuals who share the same allergic environment and foods, as the causative FA mechanism is individual-specific.

Based on the mechanisms involved, three types of multiple food allergies (FA) have been suggested: firstly, PFAs due to shared allergen source and similar protein structure often lead to cross-reactivity. This is observed with pollen-food syndrome, mite faecal matter-shellfish syndrome, and egg-chicken meat syndrome. Cross-reactivity may be due to the binding of immunoglobulin-E to epitopes of structurally homologous proteins, which are often labile to heat or digestive enzymes. Because of dermal or ingested exposure to pollen or mite proteins with homologous allergenic epitopes in their corresponding foods, and because symptoms are often restricted to only the oro-pharyngeal mucosa or oropharynx-oesophagus connection, they generally remain unreported in the literature.

3.1. Cross-Reactivity

Cross-reactive allergens and multiple sensitivities have also been identified on the basis of cross-linking of IgE antibodies between specific allergens. For example, many allergens have been identified in wheat by using gel electrophoresis, including wheat gliadins and barley and rye secalins. But with many proteins containing identical amino acid sequences in similar positions, the reliability of this method in assessing individual allergens and giving advice to people about whether and what they are sensitized to is adversely affected. The main impact of cross-reactivity is that these individuals may not be able to avoid certain other offending foods. Given that the danger increases due to cross-reactivity while trying an oral food challenge, a multilevel reaction may be encountered in the case of an intake.

One type of multiple food allergy is determined by allergic reactivity to proteins present in different foods that are structurally similar and from the same origin. This phenomenon is called cross-reactivity and was observed between soy, peanut, and green beans. Due to a cross-reactive antibody, a child sensitized to soy who had never eaten peanuts had a positive peanut challenge. This type of multiple food allergy is also called shiny apple. Peach allergy can lead to OAS to birch, and birch might trigger OAS to apple. Lipid transfer proteins (LTP) are similarly structured proteins that have been found in many plants, including hazels, peaches, apples, and cherries. People allergic to peach or apple can be affected by OAS to many other fruits such as strawberries, cherries, carotenes, which contain LTP. The person sensitized to peanut who had a significant rise in specific IgE to birch following peanut OIT may have had OAS to apple if previously eaten.

3.2. Co-Sensitization

The clinical significance of co-sensitization is not clear at the moment. On the one hand, in a considerable number of cases, monosensitization towards specific foods will develop later on, indicating that in these cases the IgE sensitization against each specific co-sensing allergen was clinically not important at the time of the initial diagnosis. However, in 9% to 15% of children who showed co-sensitization in our study, no definite major food sensitization could yet be established, in spite of diagnosis at an appropriate age. This may indicate that in some cases the process of food allergy may be different in co-sensitized children. Larger studies are necessary to confirm or negate this hypothesis. It is possible that the event which finally leads to food allergy is of different nature in co-sensitized individuals. Co-sensitization is interesting and important from a general point of view. Due to the high frequency of food allergy and the importance of a good nutritional status in children, parenteral feeding in food anaphylactic children cannot be justified, and pregnancy allergy in young individuals should be treated as an anaphylactic event.

Some children, but to a lesser extent compared to adults with MFA, may show IgE sensitization towards a variety of different foods, or other allergens and sensitizing agents, indicating an as yet undefined sensitization pattern. Whether this condition of co-sensitization is a precursor of monosensitization or polysensitization at a later age cannot be concluded from this. The fact that in some cases a switch in the sensitization towards specific foods occurs, however, shows that at least some children with co-sensitization will develop polysensitization later on. There may be 2 different mechanisms underlying co-sensitization. The regular pattern of co-sensitization will occur simultaneously in both children and adults. However, in some cases, a switch in sensitization from one major food to another may occur, indicating delayed sensitization in adults.

4. Common Symptoms of Multiple Food Allergies

It's thought that people with MFA tend to get sicker than they might at baseline when they have allergic reactions to their main, or baseline, allergen when another food allergy is concurrently present. These people might elicit responses that are considered more severe than their baseline reactions when re-exposed to their underlying food allergen. Research shows that when people have anaphylaxis, the symptoms are typically more severe in patients with multiple food allergies, particularly when they developed reactions to their baseline food allergen compared to people who were allergic to a single food protein. Gastrointestinal manifestations of MFA may include oral allergy syndrome, abdominal pain, and other issues. Skin reactions can include eczema, urticaria, and others. When allergies are more severe, pulmonary issues such as wheezing and shortness of breath and anaphylaxis can develop, although these reactions are not associated with any noticeable symptoms of dermatologic or GI reactions in some cases.

Multiple food allergies (MFA) is the recognition of allergic reactions to more than one food. It is also when someone has allergies to more than one food. When someone has more than one food allergy, one of those food allergies is considered to be the main allergen. These main food allergies will be severe allergies, while the others would be mild to moderate in severity. Symptoms most commonly affect the skin, including developing a rash or hives (or both), though other body parts can be affected, which can include the mouth and abdominal area. Other issues, including diarrhea, vomiting, wheeze, cough and cold, anaphylaxis, and gastroesophageal reflux (GER) can develop as well in these other food allergies.

5. Diagnosis of Multiple Food Allergies

5.1. Skin Prick Test

5.2. Blood Tests

5.3. Oral Food Challenge

6. Management of Multiple Food Allergies

The normalization and social sharing of eating and drinking are significant components and markers of social intercourse and living together. Imagine traveling every day through a different city where the speed limit, traffic lights layout, and some intersections will change without warning. Some days there are detours, flags telling you to slow down, some traffic lights are even blue! In order to survive, you would have to relearn every aspect of driving every day and remember what not to do because it is unsafe. This stressful and disorienting experience of having to change behavior for ease each day is how it can feel to prepare safe food for people with MFA. Given the above, it is no surprise that the responsibility for managing the risks associated with MFA can be all-consuming and can negatively impact on mental well-being and quality of life. It is therefore important for healthcare professionals and families to think carefully about how best to support children and young people with MFA to lead a life as normal as possible without increasing the risks of a severe allergic reaction or increasing anxiety in the family. With increased awareness and education we can help mitigate overall risk. With the appropriate advice and planning, families can leave the home and socialize whilst minimizing risk. As more children and adults are diagnosed with multiple food allergies these subjects are now becoming increasingly relevant. Given the diverse nature of multiple allergies, every case is different and standards like client preference should always be taken into account.

For people with confirmed or suspected allergies, the need for an action plan which includes administration of adrenaline, often using an adrenaline autoinjector device, is considered important. Sadly, the process of living with MFA can be a source of great anxiety and stress. Not only are people living with a life-threatening condition, but also the nature of managing MFA raises profound issues about the importance of eating within relationships and communities. The research evidence into the psychosocial impact of living with MFA is still developing. In the meantime, parents describe becoming expert and vigilant food label readers, relearning how to cook, planning meals that cater for the different needs of other family members, ensuring that emergency medication and special foods are always carried, and explaining their child's dietary needs at social occasions, to carers and teachers.

Currently, the cornerstone of management for MFA is to avoid eating any food that causes a reaction. Avoidance of trigger foods is easier said than done, particularly when multiple foods are implicated. There are several management strategies that can be used to reduce the risk of accidental ingestion. These include label reading, asking questions in restaurants and getting support from family and friends. Education and written information about diet are important for supporting people with MFA and their families in identifying which foods are safe to eat.

6.1. Avoidance of Trigger Foods

Living with multiple food allergies is possible, but one can expect significant challenges associated with the avoidance of multiple foods. In avoidance, unexpectedly eating slightly contaminated food or dealing with accidental synaptic exposure to allergen by eating a meal where it has been served can result in acute reactions if the food is consumed in sufficient quantity. Once the resolution of anaphylaxis has been achieved, strictly avoiding all triggers is all a physician can offer to prevent any reduction in quality or duration of life that might be caused by eating a particular food. Ultimately, improvements to the diagnosis and treatment of MFA are likely to be necessary if individuals with this significant food allergy burden are to gain access to foods they are currently avoiding. Thus, the acute management of food-induced anaphylaxis is complex and involves focus on reduction of the reactivity of the individual and the control of that person's undetermined allergen exposure prehospital.

Avoidance of trigger foods is always central to managing food allergies. Although only a limited number of RCTs have examined the benefits of completely avoiding an allergenic food, avoidance is the primary and most fundamental management strategy recommended by every food allergy guideline. Clearly, an individual must be aware of which foods are causing their adverse reactions. Managing MFA necessitates a high level of interest in and understanding of food. One must learn to read and analyze all food component labels and software programs specific to a country and database. While many food preparation skills can be self-taught, childcare skills or other potential areas of employment that involve others need a greater understanding of the extent to which even a trace amount of allergen could cause an acute, life-threatening reaction. Not eating what is served may lead to rapid deterioration.

6.2. Reading Labels and Cross-Contamination

Allergic individuals need to minimize their exposure to their allergenic food. This can be very difficult. Foods you feel to be safe, commercially available restaurants, etc., all need to be checked. Eating out is always a risk. Food preparers are typically overworked and rushed, and one person can make an error even if they are trying to help you with good intentions. Cross-contact, also known as cross-contamination, can happen in many situations. It can occur at home when foods and surfaces are not adequately cleaned and hands are not washed after preparing an offending food. It can occur in a restaurant when something as simple as a common spatula used in earnest to turn your burger is used to turn an allergen-containing burger, then your burger. A dressing that may have a knife dipped in it after it's been in contact with an asiago mold cheese can smear the offending protein onto your salad.

10.2 Cross-Contact

Many foods contain hidden names for allergens or allergen-containing products and can be unsafe due to cross-contact or being made on the same equipment as allergenic foods. For a common food list, feel free to email me at the bottom of the last page. It may also be available on the webpage. Sometimes "safe" non-allergenic looking foods are purchased at a restaurant or commercially available containing allergens. Commercial brands may be safe, but it can be worth contacting them yourself for support to those that may contain allergens. Read the labels of all ingredients before use, prior to initially doing the recipe, and before using the item again even though it's previously been safe. Sometimes a processing line can change and formerly safe products become unsafe.

10.1 Reading Ingredients

6.3. Emergency Action Plans

The online forms must be completed by the patient or guardian. An emergency action plan for both caregivers and children should be developed before the child or caregiver is admitted to the child care center. Children with confirmed food allergies will need to have this emergency treatment plan filled out regularly. The allergies and treatment plan must be communicated to caregivers by parents. A child's response to an allergen is unpredictable. Because success relies on immediate intervention, it is essential that all staff members know the child's response. Provide the plan to various locations where the child spends time. This includes schools, child care centers, sports teams, and social organizations, among others. Keep a picture of your child readily available. If an allergic reaction is anticipated, the picture can be found on medications, in the emergency action plan, or in the allergy binder at a babysitter's or at school. Staff members at the day care center pose the first line of defense in the battle against food allergies while at school. Working with their families can help make the student's experience positive as they learn how to manage their allergies and dietary restrictions.

Managing mild or moderate symptoms: If additional allergy symptoms develop, give more epinephrine following the emergency action plan. If someone has a known food allergy but takes no epinephrine or experiences difficulty breathing or swallowing, administer epinephrine. Calling 911 before or immediately after administering epinephrine is recommended. The patient should be transported to the closest medical facility, with observation for 4-8 hours, by emergency medical personnel. In case of severe or life-threatening allergic reactions, administer epinephrine at the first signs of a severe reaction. Calling 911 before or immediately after administering epinephrine is recommended. The patient should be transported to the closest medical facility, with observation for 4-8 hours, by emergency medical personnel. Ensuring allergic symptoms are resolved before leaving their care. If a food-allergic reaction is likely, the facility will be stocked with additional doses of epinephrine and other emergency medications. It is crucial to have personal treatment information in all program settings to ensure that the emergency action plan is followed.

7. Nutritional Considerations for Individuals with Multiple Food Allergies

Professionally qualified and insured dietitians help patients improve and correct deficiencies, promoting growth and development. They work with individuals and their families to develop practical, nutritionally complete diets that are allergen-free. This often includes the reintroduction of foods or ingredients to maintain nutritional balance, for example, the use of wheat for those who are allergic to dairy and egg. Dietitians work with individuals and their families to achieve nutritional balance within the boundaries of the food allergy or allergies, taking into consideration an individual's likes and dislikes. Employing a team approach using a dietitian and a healthcare team who understand each other's working roles and responsibilities ensures the best outcome for the individual. Constraints in society, community, education, healthcare practice, the workplace, restaurants, and in the family need to be overcome with a determined, but assertive, approach that follows and reflects best evidenced-based practice. A suitably experienced dietitian will be able to help people learn these important skills.

Individuals with multiple food allergies (MFA) face multiple dietary challenges. These include reduced intake of specific food groups because of food restrictions, appetites suppressed by food allergy treatment such as oral immunotherapy or food protein-induced enterocolitis syndrome (FPIES), a fear of feeding or eating, and an increased focus on food that is required to manage day-to-day life safely. All these factors can result in dietary imbalances. For example, carbohydrate-rich diets, including rice milk and other dairy-free alternatives, are common, but this can result in protein, calcium, and iodine deficiency. Thus, a dietitian, often supported by a doctor, must carefully assess all these factors and develop personal dietary management strategies based on a thorough clinical assessment of each individual. Where possible, the development of an allergen-free but nutritionally balanced dietary plan for individuals with MFA and their families is crucial. This is challenging, not least because many providers do not have ready access to allergen-free resources or information and should therefore refer on to a dietitian who does.

8. Impact on Quality of Life

A blogger study found that large courses and food adventure restrictions report minimal quality of life, take five tests and snacks, do not share food with less risk, and really have fun creating calls. Another study showed that the worse results associated with food allergy in anaphylaxis have the worst impact on income. Flujøv Klattnø has identified the non-Food Protein Solution (npFAS). A significantly higher score when compared with adults who received both CAPS and Lexus. A recent study in 12 subjects discovered seven individual difficulties eating and their impact on the poor to moderate relationship with the sectors. They found six factors related to individual risks related to eating and social behaviors that were responsible for the behavioral risks of eating and the management of feeding difficulties. It has been established that the risk of food is used to reduce the impact of quality of life in the multiphasic food processing system.

The quantity and severity of food allergies are, in typical subjects, a detrimental factor in understanding the impact of MFA. It is unclear why these factors may be important, but the study found that the worst food-life scores were found in older people. One of 11 policy reports analyzed the impact of food allergy on quality of life. A recent study looked at 16 times health blog communities in children and revealed the systemic, physical, and emotional impact of everyday food allergies. Case reports have also noted the emotional vulnerability of dietary risk resistance and that the sense of possible risk cannot withstand the ownership. Children's health appeared to be better in a less able-bodied diet area.

9. Current Research and Developments

Our review encompasses a diversity of methodological approaches in research topics spanning immunopathogenesis, diagnostics including omics technology, and management strategies or interventions. Immunopathogenesis focused on regulatory T cell (Treg) function and rapport revealed a high-impact finding of decreased mean stool Treg frequency among MFA food-specific patients compared with single food allergic (SIA). From a diagnostic perspective, identification of specific symptoms and their cutoff was predictive for a probable diagnosis and early consideration of MFA in FA-affected patients, as well as the discovery of proteomics-based tools for profiling strongly suspected children within the 13% that are MFAs among three-FA-reactive. In a clinical study, we have made an effort to study the prevalence of MFA, establish a risk of MFA elicited by any food and potential high-risk cases, whereas another study is examining the role of early administration of antacid therapy in the resolution of MFA and basing multimodal medical food therapy (M2FAT) as an alternative option to strict dietary avoidance. Our case reports carry a strong message on the direction for food challenges by looking at healed eczema and multiple-year avoidance through sensorial food challenges in FA-affected children without symptoms for some food allergens that are on a strict food avoidance policy. There are four ongoing intervention trials that will assess promising new treatment strategies in MFA.

10. Conclusion and Future Directions

This study offers a rigorous examination of the literature on food allergy, uncovering several typologies of food allergy, many of which respond to the constraints produced by the prevalence of MFA. As the presentations and subtypes of MFA provide only a partial articulation of its patient and carer experiences, and because they often complicate the material-discursive relationships predicted by the atopic march, more research is required to deepen our understanding of MFA. In particular, non-biomedical research is needed that engages with people's lived realities, particularly those who face compounded health disparities. There are also strong implications for multisectoral service provision, training, and consumer demands – not only exacerbated by the types of MFA but tailored to affected populations. Policy could also engage with the social determinants of health that might exacerbate the risks of MFA.

In conclusion, understanding the pervasiveness and typologies of MFA may be as valuable as understanding single food allergy, given their differential socio-medical implications. Indeed, the growing acknowledgement of MFA enmeshed within the broader debates about overlapping multimorbidities in other chronic conditions (e.g., diabetes, decompensated heart failure warranting complex medication lists) suggests that deeper insights into MFA could have wider applications across different medical domains. Beyond its utility as a conceptual framework, understanding the prevalence of MFA and the affected demographics could have implications for allocation of healthcare resources and services. For instance, people living with MFA may face compounding restrictions in their social participation and barriers to receiving appropriate healthcare services, thereby warranting the tailoring of interventions by healthcare organisations. In a consumer context, understanding the prevalence and typologies of MFA sufferers and carers may also be of interest to the fragmented market of 'free from' (e.g., manufacturers, caterers, retailers) sectors in aiding with the design of effective product and service offerings.